Healing Herbs:

Top 20 Medicinal Herbs to Growing, Harvesting, and Using

Table of content

Introduction

To begin, this book gives a broad manual about the use of herbs, which can be utilized for therapeutic purposes. Herbs have been utilized for healing purposes since a very long time. Therefore, it is important to provide a detailed manual regarding the use of herbs as medicines. Besides, this book covers different perspectives about herbs and their uses in the field of pharmaceutical.

Firstly, the book portrays the herbs which can be utilized for cooking and therapeutic purposes. These herbs are valuable in reinforcing the body functioning and additionally, recuperating the sicknesses. Furthermore, the herbs which can be utilized to improve the personality are incorporated in this book. These herbs are utilized as skin and hair cares. In addition, by utilizing these items, you will watch a sudden gleam in your skin and an improved hair texture. Thirdly, herbs to cure normal infirmities are incorporated. These herbs are useful in curing numerous sicknesses e.g. fever and influenza.

Another significant part of this book is the consolidation of those herbs, which are used to cure pain and itchiness. Finally, the restorative herbs for toothache are incorporated to encourage the client. This will help the client in killing toothache in case of crisis. Subsequently, this book is a finished guide for restorative herbs.

Thus, after you have read this book, you can cure numerous ailments by utilizing natural ingredients. These cures incorporate the utilization of herbs that can be developed at home.

Chapter 1 – Best Herbs to Grow for Cooking and Medicinal Use

Growing herbs in your own house is one of the most efficacious hobbies. Since it is not only money saving hobby, but also, a fun activity; therefore, many people recommend adopting this kind of productive hobby. Moreover, with the help of this hobby, you can ensure clean and healthy food for you and your family. In addition, herbs are a rich source of antioxidants; thus, they are extremely essential in everyday food. When a person consumes herbs, which are rich source of antioxidant, they react with the free radicals and make sure of body safety.

Another important aspect of the home-grown vegetables and herbs is that they are fresh and thus rich in nutrients. It is considered that the herbs lose their nutritional value after thirty minutes of their harvest. However, when you have your own fresh herbs, you can use them whenever you desire, thus your herbs will possess high nutritional value. In addition, numerous herbs are extremely useful in curing certain common illness. Therefore, it is a smart choice to grow herbs in your own house. These herbs will help you in cooking as well as in medicinal use.

Following are some of the commonly grown herbs which are efficient for cooking purposes and medicinal use:

Rosemary:

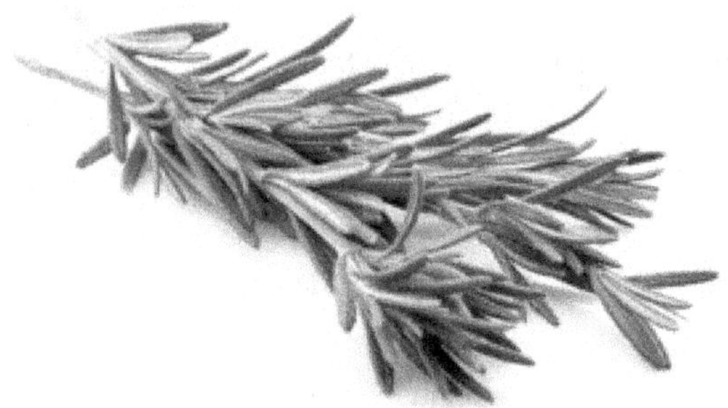

Rosemary is a pretty and aromatic herb with many nutritional elements. Rosemary contains caronsic acid, which possess the quality to cure carcinogenic cells. Moreover, the fragrance of rosemary is used to improve the memory of individuals.

How to harvest:

In order to harvest and grow rosemary, adopt the following procedure:

- To begin, plant rosemary cutting in a pot with sand one third of peat moss in it.

- Rosemary does not need to be watered frequently neither it demands a lot of fertilizers. Therefore, use moderate amount of fertilizers and water.

- Trim the plant as per the requirement.

Uses of rosemary:

Rosemary is an essential herb, which is used to cure numerous body problems. Due to the presence of numerous nutrients, rosemary is used in food as well as in medicines. Some of the uses of rosemary are as follows:

- Rosemary is used along with the oil to eradicate irritation and itchiness. Therefore, it is among one of the herbs, which are used when a person suffers from eczema and arthritis.

- Moreover, when rosemary is used externally, it cures bruises and wounds within a small time interval.

- Rosemary is further used in repelling small pests like mosquitoes. Therefore, they are often employed in the green areas where a lot of pests are found.

Thyme:

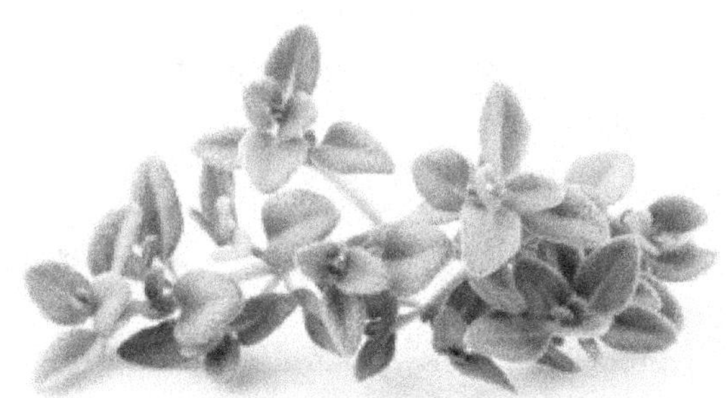

Thyme is a delicate yet an aromatic herb, which is rich source of iron and vitamins. Dried as well as fresh thyme is used for many purposes because of its nutritional value. They possess great importance since they can be incorporated in various dishes along with egg as well as the vegetables. They have elliptical, curly leaves which small width. The lower side of thyme is white in color; however, the upper part is green-grey in color.

How to harvest:

In order to harvest and grow thyme, adopt the following procedure:

-       To begin, plant thyme in summers using leaves along with sprigs.

-       Water them properly to improve their growth.

-       Thyme can be used as it is or it can be dried.

Uses of thyme:

This white colored herb is often used by many herbal doctors to cure diseases. Moreover, it has emerged to be a favorite of many people because of its effectiveness. Some of the uses of thyme to cure common pains and diseases are as follows:

-       Thyme is used to regulate the blood pressure. This can be effective when you replace the salt in your food with thyme. By doing this, you will not only regulate your blood pressure, but also, you will able to manage your cholesterol.

-       Thyme is utilized in order to improve the immunity system of the body. Because of the presence of Vitamin A and Vitamin C in thyme, they can help you fight diseases.

- Thyme is further used to disinfect your surroundings. In order to meet the purpose, use thyme oil and get rid of many infectants e.g. mols.

Basil:

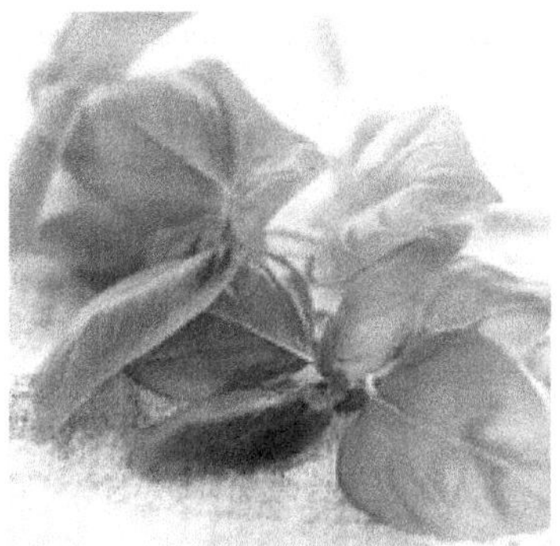

Basil is an important herb since it contains Vitamin K and volatile oils. Basil's oils and the flavonoid are efficacious in providing special health benefits; therefore, it must be utilized with various food items. Since they contain an aroma, which is admired by a lot of people therefore, it has become a part of food including pasta, omelet and curry.

How to harvest:

In order to harvest and grow basil, adopt the following procedure:

- To begin, harvest the basil using some leaves in fall.

- Plant them outdoor and water them.

- Collect all your basil leaves before the first snow fall.

Uses of basil:

Basil is extremely important herb, which is used to produce many health benefits. This herb is commonly used by the people to fight common ailments. Moreover, it is also used in food and beverages to enhance taste. Some of the uses of Basil are included in the following text:

- Basil is used to calm the stomach pain. When a person suffers from stomach ache, a basil tea is served to him to calm down the ache.

- In case a person got stung by a bee or anything, he can use basil leaves to cure them. By chewing some basil leaves or even by applying them on the effected region, the person will feel relieved.

- Basil leaves can further be used to reduce stress. In order to fulfill the purpose, soak them in warm water and drink that water. Moreover, arrange a hot tub bath with basil leaves in it, this can also providing soothing effect.

Parsley:

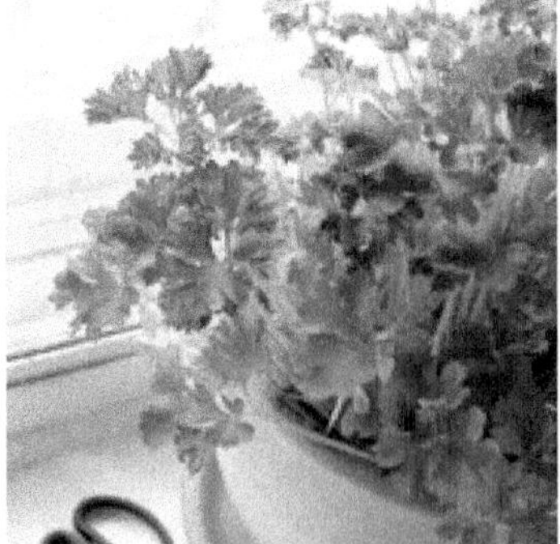

Parsley is delicious as well as very healthy in taste. Moreover, they possess healing properties, which enhance their role in food and other beverages. They are among the most popular herbs in the world because of their healing properties and aroma. Multiple people employ the use of parsley to fight flu and cold.

How to harvest:

In order to harvest and grow parsley, adopt the following procedure:

- To begin, choose young plants.

- After their stems turn green they can be used to plant.

- Cut them from the base in order to fulfill the purpose.

- Moreover, parsley can also be planted using seeds. However, seeds must be dried before planting them.

Uses of parsley:

Parsley is an extremely useful herb. It can be used in food products as well as in many beverages. Moreover, it is used to help people in fighting common ailments. Some of the uses of parsley are as follows:

- Parsley is utilized to improve health. Their volatile oils are a rich source of myristicin, which helps in improving human health.

- Parsley is an amazing anti-oxidizing agent, which reacts with the free radicals in the body and protects them from damaging any body parts. The flavonoid present in parsley, helps in eradicating oxygen based damage to the body.

-       Parsley is a great source of Vitamin C and Vitamin K. These vitamins are necessary for efficient body growth.

-       Parsley is a rich source of folic acid. Since folic acid improves the heart conditions; therefore, parsley is also used by heart patients.

Chapter 2 – Best Healing Herbs to Grow for Beauty

From the beginning of this world, herbs are being used as skin and hair cares. However, with the development of cosmetic industry, the use of herbal beauty products has faced a decline. Interestingly, the cosmetic products contain a huge portion of herbs in the ingredient list; therefore, herbs still comprise a great part of our beauty products. Since, the natural beauty products are comparatively less expensive; therefore, they can be used instead of the expensive branded beauty products.

On the contrary, skin is an extremely sensitive body organ; thus, it is essential to take care of this delicate organ. All of those things you apply on your skin became the part of your body via your body pores. Hence, the herbs you are using on your skin must be tested before their application on your skin. Moreover, not all kinds of herbs are suitable to be used on the skin. In addition to that, hair is another important part of your body. They hold the ability to either enhance your beauty, or place it to the lowest level. Many herbs are famous for their hair oils. These oils are used by many for better hair growth and hair thickness. Therefore, it is quintessential to wisely choose hair friendly herbs. Given below are some of the herbs that can be used as beauty products.

Chamomile:

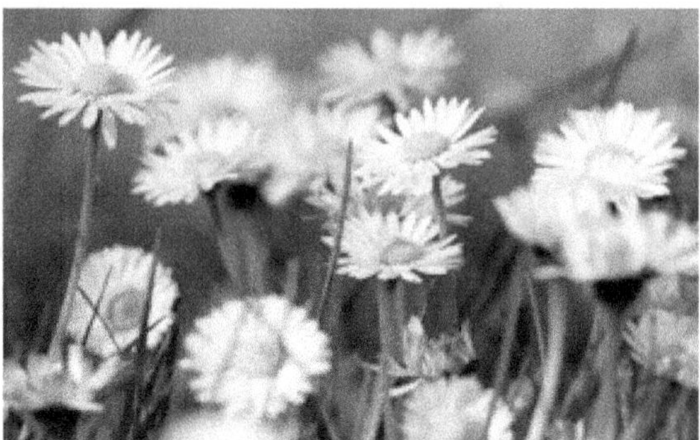

Chamomile is one of the many kinds of daisy like plants. They belong to the family of Asteraceae. Moreover, only two out of a hundred species of chamomile are used. These species are Marticaria recutita and Chamaemelum nobile. These herbs are often used for calming as well as an anti-inflammatory herb. Moreover, they have numerous other health advantages.

How to grow and harvest:

In order to harvest and grow chamomile, adopt the following procedure:

- Choose a dry day to plant chamomile. To begin, plant the stem or seed o chamomile in an average to poor soil.

- Water them properly and place them in sunlight to provide appropriate growth area.

- However, remember to plant them in a landscape and not in pots.

- Harvest them in any dry day.

Uses of chamomile:

- Chamomile is utilized as tea, which is used in case a person suffers from rheumatic problems and rashes.

- Chamomile is further used to soothe the wounds and hemorrhoids.

- Chamomile can also be used to eradicate the beginning symptoms of asthma and cold.

- Moreover, after using chamomile, the person feel relieved from restlessness and toothaches.

Neem:

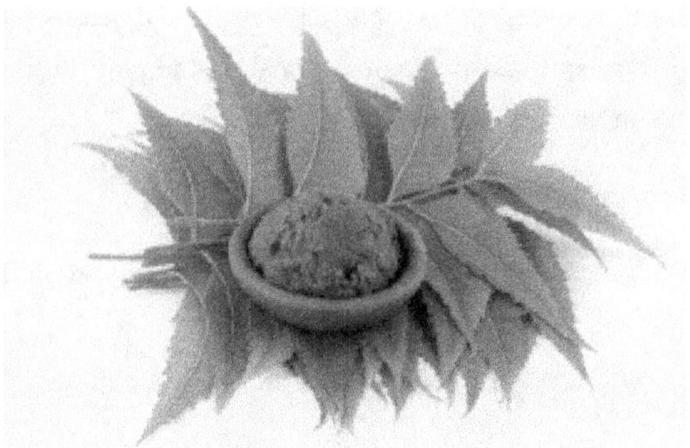

Neem is a huge herb that is commonly used throughout the year. Moreover, its height ranges up to 15 inches. Furthermore, its branches are widespread in a shape of a crown. It is used extensively because of its ability to heal and cure. Moreover, it is used in fragrances to add aroma. In addition, they have tremendous effects to improve the beauty by eradicating the body garbage. Consequently, the skin is nourished.

How to grow and harvest:

In order to harvest and grow neem, adopt the following procedure:

- Neem can be easily planted. To begin, take some neem seeds.

- Plant these seeds in a pot filled with some good mixture.

- Keep them wet and let them grow in proper sunlight.

- The neem will start germinating within a few weeks.

Uses of neem:

Neem is an extremely useful herb. It contains the ability to cure the diseases by providing a soothing effect. Moreover, it is capable of eradicating the pain in the intestine. Some of the uses of neem are as follows:

- Neem is utilized for improving the skin.

- The bark of neem is capable of curing malaria, intestinal ulcers and skin diseases.

- The neem flower is used to regulate bile and phlegm.

- Furthermore, neem is used to fight the intestinal worms.

- Neem is further used as an insecticide.

Comfry:

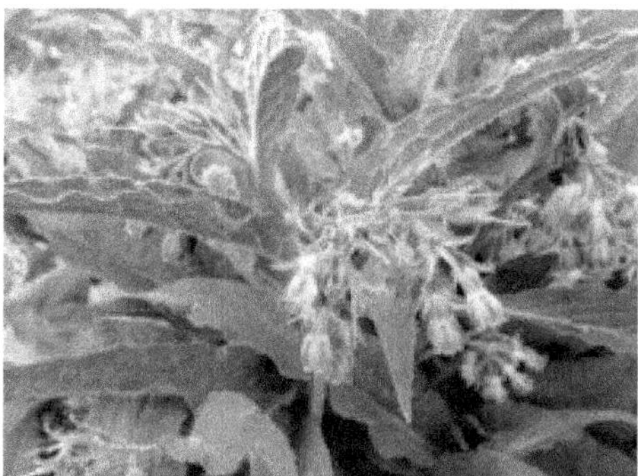

Leaves of comfrey contain high contents of moisture as well as they are dried gradually as compared to the other herbs. For better results, provide them additional time and care during their growth. Ensure the leaves are brittle before their storage; however, care must be taken as any remaining sogginess will bring about mold. At that point, pack them in the airtight containers.

How to grow and harvest:

In order to harvest and grow comfrey, adopt the following procedure:

- Start plantation in spring or fall. However, summer is also applicable for the plantation.

- Plant the seed or the stem accordingly in a wide area.

- Water them properly and maintain adequate sunlight.

- Harvest the seeds or the flowers or even the leaves, depending upon the requirement.

Uses of comfrey:

Comfrey is an important herb, with multiple uses. In order to understand its uses, consider the following points:

- Comfrey oil can effectively cure rashes. Since, it cannot be applied on deep wounds; therefore, care must be taken in case of such wounds.

- Aside from treating injuries, the oil has uses in curing the broken bones as well as the torn ligaments. Interestingly, they can be used in the body parts where you cannot put a cast

- Further, it is considered as an anti-inflammation because of its natural healing powers.

Sage:

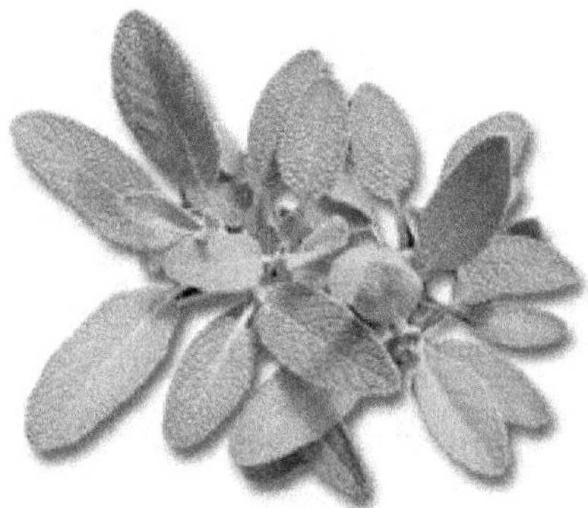

Common sage is a subshrub which is used for numerous purposes because of its ability to cure diseases and its immense healing powers.

How to grow and harvest:

In order to harvest and grow sage, adopt the following procedure:

- Sage can be grown from seeds as well as from stem cutting.

- Before the spring stars, plant the seeds in a well-drained soil.

- Water them properly and harvest the leaves or barks, as per the requirement.

Uses of sage:

This grey barked plant is extremely useful for the following purposes:

- Sage is an anti-inflammatory. Therefore, it is used to cure mouth disorders.

- It serves as a relaxant, which enhances the beauty.

- Sage reduces some of the menopausal symptoms.

Chapter 3 – Herbs for Common Ailments

The use of herbs to cure ailments dates back to about a thousand years. Numerous novel ways to treat ailments have been discovered ever since then. Moreover, even the drugs created today use the components of various plants and animals. Many healers use herbs as a drug to cure common ailments like flu, fever and hiccups. These herbs do not only cure many diseases, but also, they are easily available. Their ability to heal the diseases and strengthen the immune system has enhanced their importance. Their effectiveness can be detected from the fact that they hold the quality to heal the ailments, which are not even cured by casual dosage of pharmaceutical drugs.

Moreover, numerous people are either allergic to the drugs manufactured in industries or they doubt their impact. In addition, some people believe that these drugs have numerous side effects which cause more damage than good; therefore, they try to avoid their use. Although, the herbal medicines are not a good substitute for the drugs made in industries, yet they can be used as an alternative. These herbal medicines can help cure multiple common diseases; yet in case of serious issues, one must consult a doctor as soon as possible. Some of the herbs with medicinal properties are given below:

Aloe Vera:

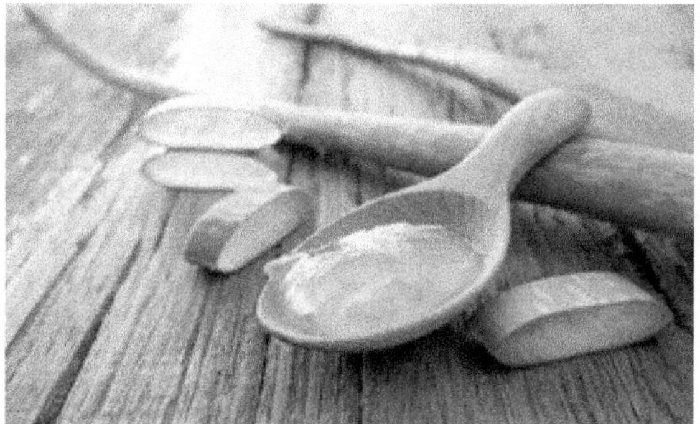

Aloe vera is an extremely useful ingredient, which cures burns along with many other problems. Therefore, it is extensively used.

How to grow harvest:

In order to harvest and grow aloe vera, adopt the following procedure:

- The baby plants of aloe are used to grow new plants.

- For that, plant them in soil which is first watered and then dried before the plantation.

- Do not water aloe excessively.

- In order to harvest, cut the leaves and extract the gel, which is used for the below mentioned purposes.

Uses of aloe vera:

- Aloe vera contains glycoproteins, which are used to cure body pain. Moreover, they eradicate inflammation as well.

- Moreover, the ability of aloe vera to repair damaged skin and tissues is derived from the polysaccharides present in it. Moreover, these polysaccharides further help in the formation of new cells.

- The lidocaines of aloe vera are very important as well. They serve as an anesthetic. This results in removal of heat sensation as well as pain.

- An efficient quality of aloe vera is that it has no oils, therefore any irritation or oiliness does not occur on the skin. Therefore, pores are not clogged on the skin.

Eucalyptus:

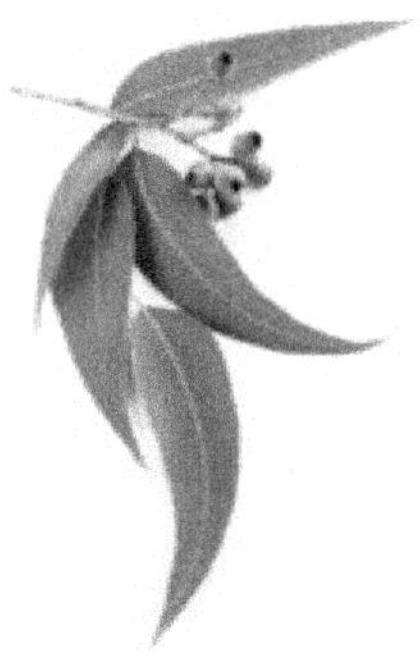

Eucalyptus is a widely used herb to eradicate pains and inflammations. It possesses a wonderful flavor and taste.

How to grow and harvest:

In order to harvest and grow eucalyptus, adopt the following procedure:

-    Plant the stem in a potting mix.

-    Place the pot in sunlight and water them adequately.

-    In order to harvest take the flowers or buds according to your requirement.

Uses of eucalyptus:

Eucalyptus has various uses. It is, however, mainly used to eradicate muscle tension and remove common ailments like flu and cold.

Fennel:

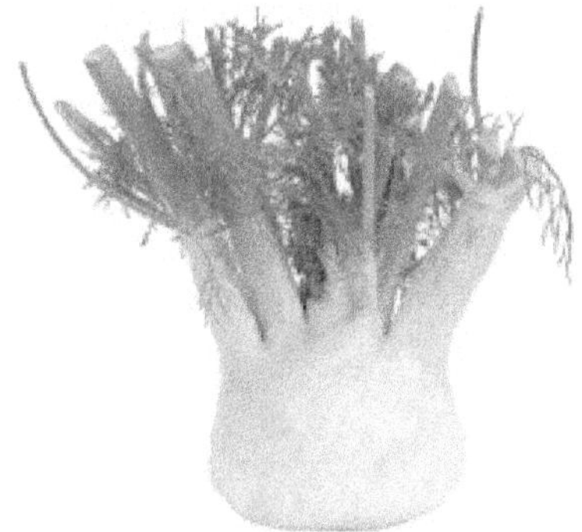

Fennel belongs to the carrot flowering family. It is used in many medicine and food items because of its healing power and nutritional value.

How to grow and harvest:

In order to harvest and grow fennel, adopt the following procedure:

- For plantation, you can either use bulbs or pre- soaked seeds.

- Plant them in the spring season and harvest when the flowers have emerged.

Uses of fennel:

Fennel is commonly used in order to eradicate pain. It provides a soothing effect on the aching muscles. In addition it is used to cure common ailments like acne and eczema.

Calendula:

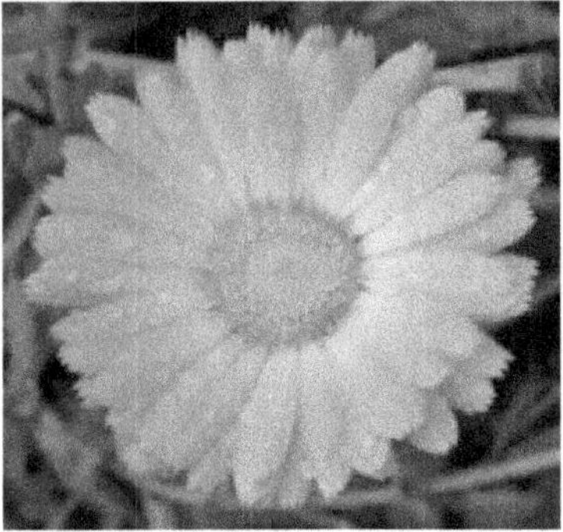

Calendula is a beautiful flower that emerges out of the stem within a short period of time. It is an extremely useful flower with healing properties.

How to grow and harvest:

In order to harvest and grow calendula, adopt the following procedure:

- Plant them using a stem or seed in a proper sunlight.

-        Water them accordingly.

-        Harvest when the flowers bloom.

Uses of calendula:

It is used for following purposes:

-        It is an anti-inflammatory.

-        It is used for natural hair coloring.

-        It is used as a diaper cream as well.

Chapter 4 – Best Herbs for Inflammation and Pain

When a person suffers from pain, of any kind, it feels like life has stopped for the sufferer. In such a situation, you prefer taking medicines with strong dosage. However, these medicines have multiple side effects which can hinder your body processing. Moreover, these medicines can also hamper your immune system. Thus, the use of herbs to cure body pain is preferred by many people.

Pharmaceutical drugs are one option to cure pain and inflammation; however, interestingly, it is not the only way. On the brighter side, multiple natural methods can be utilized for pain relief instead of strong pain-killers and prescribed drugs. Some herbs are discussed in the coming part of the chapter, which will help in curing pain and treat inflammations as well. These herbs are responsible for the generation of prostaglandins, which regulate the inflammation. Although herbs are efficient and simple to use, yet care must be taken while their utilization. Try and use the herbal creams or masks on a small portion of your skin, so that your skin is not damaged. In case of extreme pain and inflammation, it is better to consult a doctor to avoid any repercussions. Following are some of the herbs used to cure pain and inflammation:

Boswellia:

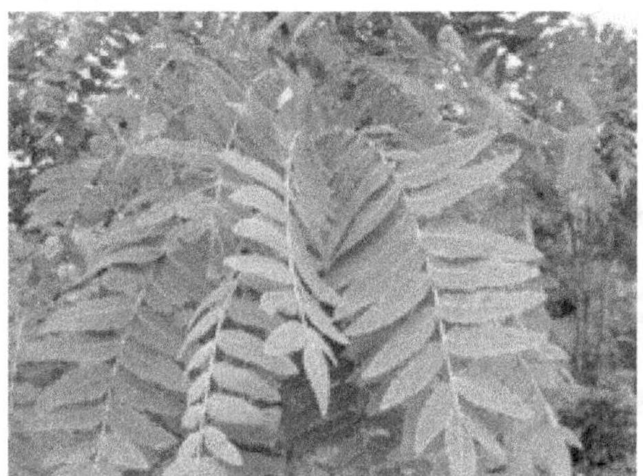

How to grow and harvest:

In order to harvest and grow boswellia, adopt the following procedure:

- Plant the stem in damp soil.

- Place them in slightly shady spots.

- Harvest when leaves become large.

Uses of boswellia:

- It cures muscles tension.

- It is an anti-inflammatory herb.

- Moreover, it can be used to eradicate intestinal cramps.

Willow bark:

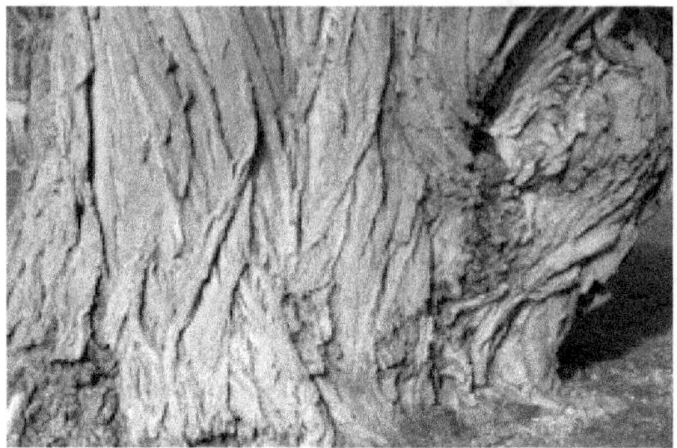

How to harvest:

Willow barks are commonly available in many parts of the world. In order to use them, cut them out of the tree barks and make small pieces of them. They are ready to be used after a slight wash.

Uses of willow bark:

Willow bark is an extremely useful bark, which has the following advantages:

-       It is used to decrease the osteoarthritis pains.

-       It eliminates acne.

-       It regulates blood pressure.

-       It is used to cure headaches.

-       Moreover, it calms the menstrual cramps.

Arnica:

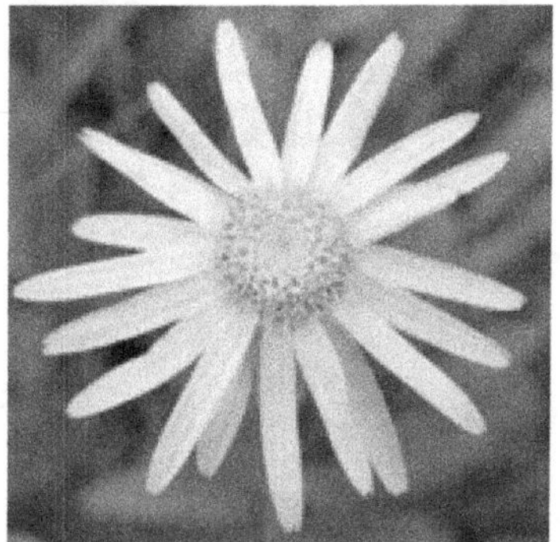

How to grow and harvest:

In order to harvest and grow arnica, adopt the following procedure:

-       Plant the stem in soil.

-       Place it in a sunny spot.

-       Water them appropriately.

-       Harvest when the flowers are ready.

Uses of arnica:

Arnica is used in order to cure the following problems:

-       It is used to remove bruises and pains.

-       It is used to control sore throats.

-       It is an anti-dandruff herb which is also used in various hair tonics.

Cayenne pepper:

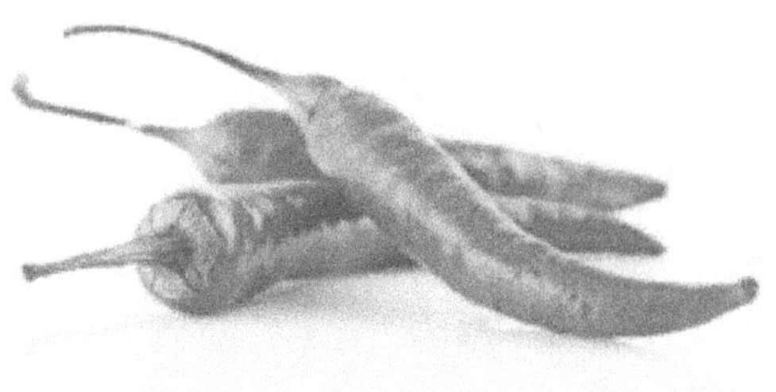

How to grow and harvest:

In order to harvest and grow cayenne pepper, adopt the following procedure:

- Plant the seeds of the pepper in a pot with soil or potting mix.

- Place them in medium sunlight spot.

- Add a lot of water, this will improve their growth.

- In order to harvest, use them as it is or you can ground them in powdered form as well.

Uses of cayenne pepper:

Cayenne pepper is used in curing the following:

- It serves as an anti-allergic.

- It is sued to cure pack pains.

- It is useful in curing blood clots.

- It cures joint pains.

Chapter 5 – Medicinal Herbs for Toothache

A toothache can be extremely painful at times; therefore, it must be cured at the fastest rate. In case a bad toothache strikes you at midnight and you are unable to reach a doctor, herbal medicines come handy at these points. Multiple herbs can be used to cure toothache at the need of the hour. These herbs do not only improve your tooth conditions, but also, strengthen your cavities.

Cavities are often caused as a result of bacteria attack on your mouth. These bacteria grow in the sugar and other food products that are stick in your teeth. Further, these bacteria produce multiple acids, which damage your teeth. Therefore, in order to eradicate the toothache, you can use numerous herbs. Some of the herbs, which can be useful in treating toothache, are incorporated in the coming text.

Cloves:

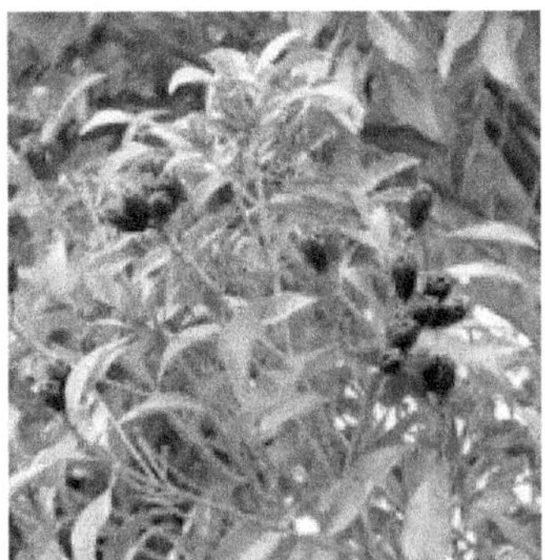

Cloves are another kind of herbs, which is commonly found and has numerous uses.

How to grow and harvest:

In order to harvest and grow cloves, adopt the following procedure:

-        In order to plant cloves, place the seed in water for a night.

-        Plant these seeds in a warm, slightly damp soil.

-        Later, when the flowers are ripened and turn purple, you can harvest the cloves.

Uses of cloves:

Following are some of the health benefits of cloves:

-        They help in overcoming toothache. When a person keeps them on the teeth, which aches then their water will provide a soothing impact.

-        Further, they are used for improved bone structure and better food digestion.

Ginger:

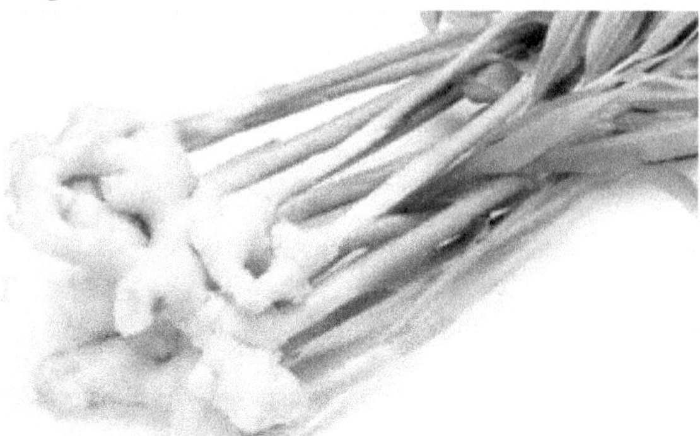

Ginger is an herb which is found commonly in all houses. It is utilized in tea and food to make them healthy. It is known to have various useful nutrients.

How to grow and harvest:

In order to harvest and grow ginger, adopt the following procedure:

-       To begin, soak the ginger roots in warm water for a night.

-       Plant these roots in a well-draining pot mixture.

-       Keep the pot slightly damp by spraying water using a spray bottle.

-       Place them in a spot, which is not directly hit by sunlight.

-       For harvesting, ginger grows under the soil.

Uses of ginger:

Ginger is famous for following purposes:

-       Chewing ginger bulbs can help reduce toothaches.

-       They are efficient in reducing stomach pains.

-       They help in curing nausea and motion sickness.

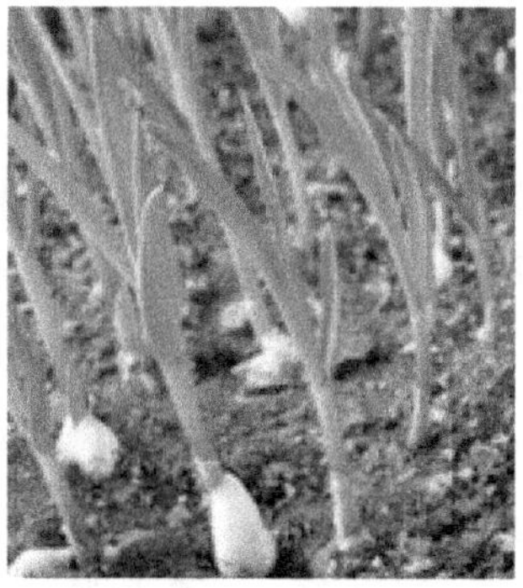

Garlic is a household ingredient, with multiple uses. It can be used to cure a lot of diseases and provide healthy imapcts.

How to grow and harvest:

In order to harvest and grow garlic, adopt the following procedure:

- Separate the garlic pieces and plant them in the late spring or fall mainly before the first frost hit the ground.

- Place them a spot which receives enough sunlight but not extra.

- Water them thrice during their growth.

- They will be ready to harvest, once they have popped out of the soil.

Uses of garlic:

Garlic is used for the following purposes:

- It is used for toothaches. One can chew garlic, in order to get rid of the pain.

- Furthermore, garlic is used to regulate the cholesterol level and the heart rate.

- They are immensely used in food item for their extensive uses.

Goldenseal:

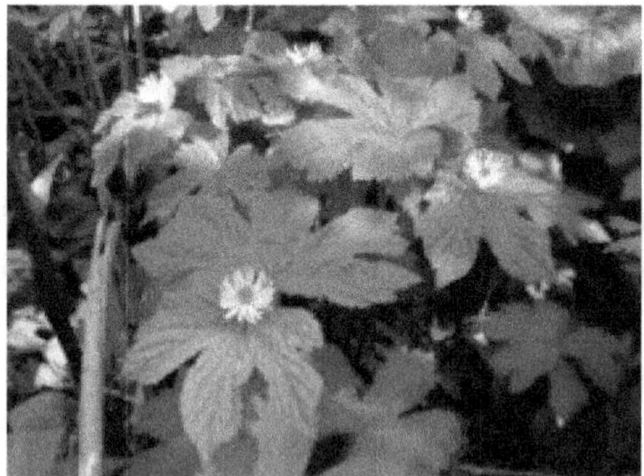

Goldenseal is an extremely useful herb, which can be used to cure toothaches and is a source of relief for many kinds of pains. Therefore, it is a good choice to be harvested at your own house.

How to grow and harvest:

In order to harvest and grow goldenseal, adopt the following procedure:

-        Sow them in a row and keep appropriate distance.

-        Plant the seeds and water them appropriately.

-        Harvest when the flower is in full bloom.

Uses of goldenseal:

-        This herb can be used to cure toothache. By chewing the herbs, one can eradicate the pain. Moreover, it can be used in a tea.

-        Goldenseal is utilized in order to cure deafness and earaches.

-        Moreover, it is used as an eye wash in case of pink eye.

Conclusion

To put in a nutshell, this book provides an extensive manual about the herbs, which can be used for medical purposes. Herbs have been used for healing purposes since a very long time; therefore, it is the need of the hour to provide a guide about the appropriate use of these herbs. Moreover, this book covers various aspects about herbs and their uses in the field of medicine.

Firstly, the book describes the herbs which can be used for cooking and medicinal purposes. These herbs are useful in strengthening the immune system as well as healing the ailments. Secondly, the herbs which can be used to enhance the beauty are included in here. These herbs are used as skin and hair cares. Moreover, by using these products, you will observe a sudden glow in your skin and an improved hair texture. Thirdly, herbs to cure common ailments are included. These herbs are helpful in curing many diseases e.g. fever, hiccups and flu.

Another major aspect of this book is the incorporation of those herbs, which are utilized in order to cure pain and inflammation. Lastly, the medicinal herbs for toothache are included to facilitate the user. This will help the user in eradicating toothache in case of emergency. Therefore, this book is a complete guide for medicinal herbs.

Consequently, after reading this book, you will be become able to cure many diseases by using natural remedies. These remedies include the use of herbs that can be grown at home.

FREE Bonus Reminder

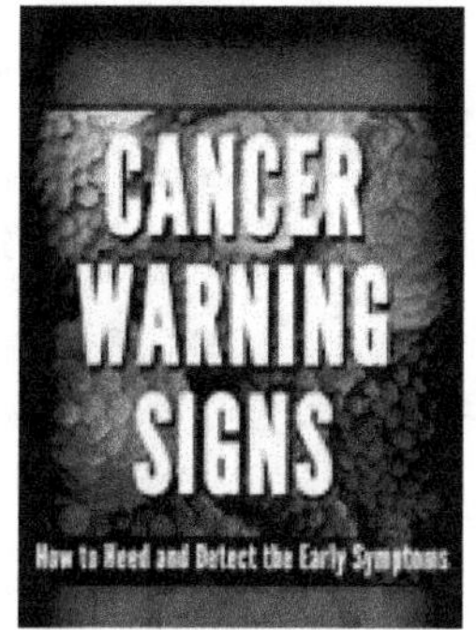

If you have not grabbed it yet, please go ahead and download your special bonus report *"DIY Projects. 13 Useful & Easy To Make DIY Projects To Save Money & Improve Your Home!"*

Simply Click the Button Below

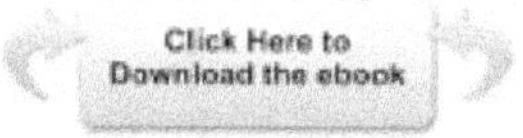

OR Go to This Page

http://healthylivingpeople.com/free/

BONUS #2: More Free & Discounted Books

Do you want to receive more Free & Discounted Books?

We have a mailing list where we send out our new Books when they go free or with a discount on Kindle. Click on the link below to sign up for Free & Discount Book Promotions.

=> Sign Up for Free & Discount Book Promotions <=

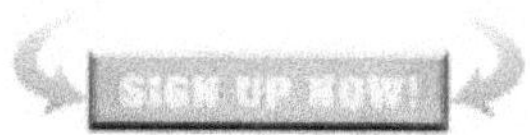

OR Go to this URL

http://zbit.ly/1WBb1Ek